Natural Sol Helicobact.. . , __ (H. Pylori)

The Complete Guide To Treatment Options, Managing Helicobacter Pylori And The Symptoms Of Helicobacter Pylori So That You Can Live A Healthy Life

Dr. Martine Nathalie

Contents

CHAPTER ONE

Helicobacter Pylori (H. Pylori)

One kind of bacteria is called Helicobacter pylori (H. pylori). Your digestive tract might become home to these bacteria after they enter your body. They may eventually lead to ulcers, which are sores that develop on the stomach or upper small intestinal lining. Stomach cancer can develop in some persons as a result of an infection.

It's typical to have an H. pylori infection. It is present in the body of about two thirds of people worldwide. Most people don't get ulcers or any other symptoms as a result of it. There are medications that can destroy the germs and speed the healing of sores if you do have issues.

Fewer people are becoming infected with the germs than in the past as more of the world gains access to clean water and sanitation. You can avoid contracting H. pylori for yourself and your kids by practicing excellent health behaviors.

How H. Pylori Causes Illness

For many years, doctors believed that ulcers were caused by stress, spicy meals, smoking, or other lifestyle choices. However, when H. pylori was identified by scientists in 1982, they found that the bacteria were the main cause of most stomach ulcers.

The lining of your stomach, which typically shields you from the acid your body produces to digest food, is attacked by H. pylori after it enters your body. Ulcers can develop once the bacteria have caused enough damage to the lining that acid can pass through. These could cause bleeding, infections, or block the passage of food through your digestive tract.

H. pylori can be acquired through food, water, or

utensils. It occurs more frequently in places or areas without good sewage or water systems. The germs can also be acquired by contact with the saliva or other bodily fluids of those who have the infection.

H. pylori is commonly acquired in children, although it can also affect adults. Although the majority of those who have it never get ulcers, the bacteria might remain in the body for years before symptoms appear. Why only certain people get ulcers after an infection is a mystery to doctors.

Symptoms

The majority of people who have H. pylori infection never experience any symptoms. Why so many people don't exhibit symptoms is unclear. However, some people might be more resistant to the negative effects of H. pylori from birth.

When H. pylori infection signs or symptoms do manifest, they are frequently linked to gastritis or a peptic ulcer and may include: • An ache or burning pain in your stomach (abdomen); • Stomach pain that may be worse when your stomach is empty; • Nausea; Loss of appetite; • Frequent burping; • Bloating; • Unintentional weight loss.

CHAPTER TWO

When To Visit A Doctor

If you experience any symptoms that could indicate gastritis or a peptic ulcer, schedule a visit with your doctor. If you have: Get emergency medical treatment.

• Constant or excruciating stomach (abdominal) pain that may cause you to wake up from sleep

• Vomit that is bloody, black, or resembles coffee grounds

Diagnosing A Problem

Your doctor won't likely perform an H. pylori test if you don't exhibit ulcer-related symptoms. But it's best to get checked if you now have them or have in the past. Since medications like nonsteroidal anti-inflammatory drugs (NSAIDs) can also harm your stomach lining, it's critical to identify the root of your symptoms in order to receive the proper care.

Your doctor will first inquire about your health history,

current symptoms, and any medications you are taking. The next step is a physical examination, which includes pressing on your stomach to feel for any swelling, discomfort, or pain. You might also:

• Blood and stool tests, which can be used to detect infections

• Breath test for urea. You will sip on a special liquid that contains urea. Then your doctor will have you breathe into a bag, which will be sent to a lab for analysis. Lab testing will reveal that your breath contains higher levels of carbon dioxide than usual if you have H. pylori, which turns the urea in your body into the gas.

Your doctor may employ the following methods to examine your ulcers more thoroughly:

Endoscopy of the upper digestive tract In a hospital, a doctor will look down your neck, into your stomach, and the top section of your small intestine using a tube with a tiny camera called an endoscope. The method can also be applied to obtain a sample that will be tested for the bacteria. Whether you are awake or sleeping throughout the surgery, you will get medication to help you feel more at ease.

• Upper GI exams You will consume a barium-containing liquid in a medical facility, and your physician will then do an X-ray on you. Your neck and stomach are plainly visible on the image thanks to the fluid that coats them.

• a CT scan, or computer tomography. It is a potent X-ray that produces in-depth images of the interior of your body.

Causes

When H. pylori bacteria infect your stomach, H. pylori infection results. The most common way for H. pylori germs to spread from one person to another is by direct contact with saliva, vomit, or stool. It's also possible for contaminated food or water to spread H. pylori. It is still unclear how the H. pylori bacterium in certain persons develops gastritis or a peptic ulcer.

CHAPTER THREE

Risk Elements

Children frequently get H. pylori infections. The following childhood living situations are associated with an increased risk of H. pylori infection: Your chance of contracting H. pylori can rise if you live in a large household.

• Lack of a consistent source of clean water. Reliable access to clean, flowing water can lower the danger of H. pylori.

• Reside in a developing nation. Infection with H. pylori is more common among residents of underdeveloped nations. This can be due to the fact that congested and unhygienic living situations are more typical in emerging nations.

• Sharing a residence with an H. pylori carrier. If you live with someone who has H. pylori infection, your chances of getting it are higher.

Complications

• Ulcers are one of the side effects of H. pylori infection. The protective lining of the stomach and small intestine can be harmed by H. pylori. This might enable stomach acid to cause an open wound (ulcer). In about 10% of H. pylori carriers, an ulcer will form.

• Stomach lining inflammation. An infection with H. pylori can irritate and inflame the stomach (gastritis).

• Gastric cancer. A significant risk factor for some kinds of stomach cancer is H. pylori infection.

Prevention

Healthcare professionals occasionally do H. pylori tests on healthy individuals in regions of the world where the virus and its consequences are prevalent. It is debatable among doctors if there is a benefit to testing for H. pylori infection when you do not exhibit any symptoms or signs of infection.

Speak with your healthcare professional if you have questions regarding H. pylori infection or believe you may be at a high risk for stomach cancer. You and your partner can determine if H. pylori testing might be beneficial for you.

What Side Effects Might H. Pylori Infections Cause?

Peptic ulcers can result from H. pylori infections, but the infection or the ulcer itself can also cause more severe consequences. These consist of:

• internal bleeding, which is linked to iron deficiency anemia and can occur when a peptic ulcer bursts through a blood artery.

• perforation, which can occur when an ulcer pierces the stomach wall; blockage, which can occur when something like a tumor prevents food from leaving your stomach;

• Peritonitis, a condition in which the peritoneum, or

lining of the abdominal cavity, becomes infected

Additionally, H. pylori can raise the risk of the stomach cancer gastric adenocarcinoma. According to a sizable cohort study published in 2019 on smokers, Black people and African Americans, Latinos and Hispanics, and Asians, this risk is increased.

Having said that, the majority of H. pylori infection sufferers never acquire stomach cancer.

CHAPTER FOUR

How Are H. Pylori Infection Treated?

Treatment may not be beneficial if you have an H. pylori infection that isn't bothering you and aren't more likely to develop stomach cancer.

H. pylori infection is linked to stomach cancer as well as duodenal and stomach ulcers. A medical expert might advise treating an H. pylori infection if you have close relatives who have stomach cancer or issues like stomach or duodenal ulcers.

An ulcer can be treated, and doing so may lower your risk of developing stomach cancer.

How Can I Avoid Contracting H. Pylori?

Although there is no vaccine to guard against H. pylori, good cleanliness and healthy habits can help avoid infection. By doing these things, you can reduce your risk of contracting H. pylori: washing your hands frequently, especially before using the restroom or when you're about to prepare or eat; drinking water from a source you know is safe; and avoiding food that hasn't been cooked or cleaned correctly.

What Can I Anticipate Down The Road?

Most H. pylori patients never show any signs of the bug or have any difficulties with it.

Your long-term prognosis is generally favorable if you are exhibiting symptoms and are receiving therapy. Your doctor will perform testing to ensure that the medication successfully eliminated the bacteria at least 4 weeks after you end your treatment. To completely eradicate the H. pylori germs, you could require more than one session of treatment.

Some persons may develop peptic ulcers as a result of H. pylori infections. A peptic ulcer may typically be healed with medical treatment for the H. pylori infection.

Your prognosis will depend on the illness, how quickly it is identified, and how it is treated if you develop another condition linked to an H. pylori infection. Very few H. pylori patients will get stomach cancer.

How Can I Avoid Getting H. Pylori?

The exact mechanism through which the bacteria spreads from person to person is unknown to health specialists. However, maintaining proper hygiene practices can keep you safe. • Washing your hands with soap and water is one of these practices. Doing this after using the restroom and before eating is crucial.

• Ensuring that the food you consume has been properly washed and prepared.

• Ensuring that the water you drink is clean and safe

Being Exposed To H. Pylori

Follow up with your healthcare professional once you've established with certainty that you have H. pylori. To ensure the bacteria have been eliminated, he or she will perform several tests.

When Should I Make A Call To My Doctor?

If your symptoms worsen or you develop new symptoms, contact your healthcare practitioner right away. If you experience signs like bloody vomit, blood in your stools, or black, tarry-looking stools, call straight away.

Major Points

Your stomach is infected with a form of bacterium called H. pylori.

• It targets the first segment of your small intestine and your stomach (duodenum). Many people with the bacteria won't show any symptoms, although it can result in redness and swelling (inflammation).

• It may be transmitted or spread from person to person by mouth, such as by kissing; • It may result in open sores in your upper digestive tract known as peptic ulcers; • It may result in stomach cancer. Additionally, it might transfer through direct touch with feces or vomit.

Next Actions

Here are some pointers to help you make the most of a visit to your doctor:

• Make a list of the questions you want answered before your visit.

• Bring a companion so you can recall what your provider tells you and to ask questions.

• While you're there, make a note of any new prescriptions, procedures, tests, or instructions the doctor provides you.

• Note the date, time, and reason for any follow-up appointments you have.

The End

Printed in Great Britain
by Amazon